Gary Toenges

NETWORK

MARKETING

Is This for You?

NETWORK MARKETING

Foreword

Do you have an Entrepreneurial spirit?

This is a journey into the world of Network Marketing, which will answer questions you may have and present a better understanding of what is involved should you venture down this road.

The folks who promote the untold riches awaiting you generally speaking are very successful in their own right. Many have achieved success in Network Marketing. They want to convince you that the same thing can happen for you.

Can It?

This is a difficult question to answer. In fact, only you can answer this!

If you have an outgoing personality, if you can sell yourself and if your fully committed in what your selling then the answer may be yes. A lot of if's is involved!

The trap many fall into is they become so caught up in the promoter's enthusiasm and perceived success that they begin to believe they too can replicate this person's success.

I joined one which I'm going to tell you about. A lot of research and investigation goes into a writing project be it a book, a report or an article. This is mine.

I formatted the pages on the paperback so you have room to make notes.

Who, What, Where, When, How & Why are the questions which need answers to come to a satisfactory conclusion in order to make an informed decision. I have done this for you and you will know at the end of this book if Network Marketing is for You.

Chapter One

<u>The pitch:</u>

What a sponsor will tell you is to give as little information as possible in the initial contact. You must engage their curiosity, intrigue them with an idea of what if. Then when the hook is set and their wanting to hear more you tell them about what you have discovered which is working for you beyond your expectations and you believe this could work for them as well.

What if, you could go back in time when Walmart or Amazon were names you had never heard of?

Yet, they were out there building their business model with hopes of creating something epic in scope and market saturation. Would you then have taken advantage of this opportunity to get in on the ground floor of one of these iconic businesses?

Amazon's IPO was priced at $18.00 per share, today it's worth over 100 times this. If you had purchased 100 shares of Walmart's IPO in 1970 after stock splits your investment today would be worth over $12 million.

What you are about to read is an opportunity like those above.

I am sending this to you because I think you will understand it and more to the point you may be interested in finding another way to supplement your income or build your own business in achieving your goal of financial security.

I was talking to my neighbor the other day, he's a Physician Assistant.

He earns a six-figure income! He told me about a side line he is working on in order to build a residual income stream as he nears retirement. He explained it to me and my first question was, "this sounds like a Pyramid scheme?"

His response, "No, it's not! This is a "Network Marketing IBO (Independent Business Owner) offering, but yes, it is what in the past were referred to as Multi-Level Marketing some of which were thought of as scams, but, MLM's/Network Marketing companies are legitimate businesses. Pyramid Schemes are illegal.

I asked my second question, "Why are you involved in this?"

His answer, "because it's easy and the work involved is not time consuming. I can work my regular job and work this as well" He then presented the facts of this business model.

Here is what got my attention; he told me that the medical schools in the U.S. teach a "Standard of Practice" which Mask & Manage conditions but that proper nutrition could correct many of the problems or put another way reset your body to cure itself!

As a Physician he must adhere to the AMA dictates of prescription medicine.

This program is a nutritional alternative in achieving good health which his education and experience knows to be true.

He confirmed to me what I already knew and what I have believed for the past fifty years (I am 70 and I take no medication whatsoever). My father lived to 94, my mother is still alive at 98. I am likely going to live for many more years and I want those years to be good ones. Staying healthy is key.

I clicked on the link he sent me after our conversation, I wanted to know why folks in the mainstream medical community who earn substantial incomes would be drawn into this.

I watched and listened with an open mind. The science behind the products for me is sound. I am in good health and in part I attribute this to staying as far away as possible from anyone associated with the American Medical Association.

In my opinion everything is a pyramid of one sort or another! Wherever you look be it Government, Corporations, Education or anything else the people at the top earn the big bucks and receive the perks their status provides them. Those under them receive much less but are doing the work.

This is the American dream working your way to the top, right? Only this dream is rarely achieved by hardworking folks like you and me.

We have been indoctrinated over the past fifty years that we must get a college degree in order to have any possible chance of getting a good paying job and achieving success. If your goal is to become a technical professional, (i.e. Doctor, Attorney, Engineer, etc.) then yes advanced education is a given.

However, to get a piece of paper that tells the world you received an education in BS is nothing more than debt enslavement. You can never flee from repaying a college loan!

Sadly, there are an untold number of people working for $15.00 an hour or less at jobs they don't want and that will not sustain a good life.

Yet they were led to believe they would have it all someday soon when they took out a student loan to get their degree.

Why am I doing this? First and foremost, I want these products for my own personal use! Secondly, not only do I receive this product for my money, I receive pre-IPO shares which will convert to stock when this company goes public. I am confident and convinced that this product will maintain or improve my good health. When the company goes public and it rises to great heights like Amazon, so much the better. Why do I think this is possible? Because the folks behind this company are rich and they wouldn't be in this if they didn't believe it will make them even richer.

There's a saying here in Texas, "Don't Mess with Texas" you'll see it on signs everywhere across the state. Well you don't want to mess with Texans either. So, here is one thing to consider, this is a Texas based company located in Frisco, Texas. Businesses here are strictly monitored by the Texas Attorney General. Additionally, this company is regulated by the FTC (Federal Trade Commission).

When you watch this, (video link inserted) you'll know if you're interested or not!

At the very least you'll come away with a different perspective on how to look at your life and hopefully make better decisions for yourself and your loved ones.

I believe from the research I have done up to now and which I will continue with, I have to conclude this could be a life changing opportunity!

<u>The Follow-Up:</u>

I will share this with you.

Phil Knight, the co-founder of Nike Shoes is one of the partners in this business. It began doing business in 2008. He cashed out of Nike a couple of years ago. Forbes states Mr. Knight, as the 28th richest man in the World.

I think you're interested in finding a way to achieve your goal of financial independence.

I use these products! I receive pre-IPO shares which will convert to stock when the company goes public. And, I believe the company is going to take off. The folks behind this company are rich and they wouldn't be in this if they didn't believe it will make them even richer.

Watch these video links, (video links inserted) you'll know if this is something you can get behind and make a business of!

This is your opportunity to become an Independent Business Owner without the burden of stocking inventory, taking orders, shipping orders or collecting money.

It's $25 for an annual membership if all you want is the product.

This is a Network Marketing company. There is no cap on what you can earn, but YOU have to do the work to make it work for you!

<u>The Personal Appeal:</u>

Emily,

This may not interest you, but I will share this with you because this is a perfect fit for your abilities and ambition. If you feel this is intrusive of me, I apologize.

I believe you could easily be making an impressive six-figure income in the next few years if you chose an opportunity with the capability of producing the kind of income you can make with this company.

The kind of income which can create a seven-figure net worth.

The old adage, "give a man a fish feed him for a day. Teach him to fish and feed him for lifetime." Well, you appear to know how to fish.

I'm asking that you watch the five videos in the link below and seriously consider the possibilities. I can visualize you doing these videos at some point in the future if your so inclined.

https://www.youtube.com/playlist?list=PL4MFPhuOCYHstZuk9HwxrvBmBK531HqtA

If you endorse good health, proper nutrition and a holistic approach to health issues major or minor then these videos will resonate with you.

Phil Knight, the co-founder of Nike is one of the partners in PURE. He cashed out of Nike a couple of years ago and has focused on new ventures. Forbes states Mr. Knight, as the 28th richest man in the World. He is providing an opportunity for regular people to achieve their own financial freedom.

I am sending this to you because I think you will understand it and more to the point you may be interested in finding another way to build your own business and achieving your goal of financial freedom.

Your Millennial generation are online buyers, they are rapidly changing their shopping habits away from brick & mortar store fronts. They are also more health savvy than past generations. My generation (Baby Boomers) are figuring out that main stream medicine has not been all that we were led to believe. The side effects in many cases are worse than the prescribed treatment. Generation X are the lost folks, between the Boomers and the Millennials. Their conflicted by what they learned growing up and confused that those teachings aren't working today.

I have watched and listened with an open mind to a number of videos on this company and testimonials on the products.

The science behind these products for me is sound.

This could become a very lucrative product line for your business. For as little as $25 you can buy a membership and join this company purchasing this product line at a discounted price. One of the products I have been using with great results is "GoYin."

There are thirty-five different products in this line of health supplements which represent value and a competitive pricing structure when compared to the national health food supermarkets or any of the one-off health direct sales companies doing business today in the U.S.

Additionally, they now have a skin care line as well.

This company is doing business in Canada, Australia, South Korea, Japan, Thailand and the United States. The company is on track to hit one Billion dollars in sales by 2020. To put this in perspective a Billion dollars is a fractional amount of business in the health industry which means the potential is realistic that it can attain a trend of grand growth in the next few years.

Why am I doing this? First and foremost, I use these products! Secondly, not only do I use this product, I receive pre-IPO shares which will convert to stock when this company goes public (projected in 2020). I believe this company is going to take off. Why do I think this? Because the folks behind it are extremely rich and they wouldn't be in this if they didn't believe it will make them even richer.

Regulated by the FTC (Federal Trade Commission). They are located in Frisco, Texas, just north of Dallas.

This is an opportunity to become an Independent Business Owner without the expense or work of stocking inventory, taking orders, shipping orders or collecting money.

It's $25 for an annual membership if all you want is the product at wholesale cost. A membership and a $75 order are what you spend on dinner and a movie. Isn't it worth it to take a chance on a product that might improve a condition you have or that someone close to you has?

This is a Network Marketing company. There is no cap on what you can earn, but YOU have to do the work to make it work! Network Marketing companies are legitimate businesses. The Author of "Rich Dad Poor Dad" endorses this path.

There is not a shortage of naysayers when the subject of network marketing is discussed. However, what's their advice and will it help you achieve what it is you really want?

I joined this company because it was the most cost-effective way for me to acquire the product. The use of the product is my priority. The business aspect has intrigued me and being retired I have been looking for something to keep me productive which I can do on my own terms.

The reality is this, the program has worked for many folks. However, Robert Kiyosaki the author of "Rich Dad Poor Dad" explains it best in the you-tube video I have included in the five videos.

The bottom line, success depends on an Entrepreneurial spirit, a desire to control your own Destiney and the strength of a self-starter. You have all three!

This is a great product line which you can promote or use or help others with in complete confidence.

Do not do this because I'm doing it! Do it because it feels right to you, that you can see the potential to achieve your own personal goals.

I think if you are looking for an opportunity to create another income stream this could be it.

Trust your instincts.

All the Best,

Gary

US11293656 is my referral number.

This link will take you to the product catalog, (add link here).

Postscript;

If you've stayed with me to the end of this letter Emily, then I think we should talk. I'm new to this as well, but, my neighbor (the

Physician Assistant) has been in this for six weeks now and has recouped his initial investment. He was convinced this works because of Brig Hart (google him) who is a big name in Network Marketing. NM has been very lucrative for him over the past years. He has been involved in many Multi-Level Marketing (Network Marketing) companies. Knowing Mr. Hart is in this brought my neighbor into this company.

Chapter Two

It's been said, "there's no such thing as bad publicity!" If your being written about or talked about your name is out there.

Network Marketing draws in a diverse cross section of people. There are no geographic restrictions and no demographic limitations.

From all walks of life and every social economic class who have achieved financial freedom in Network Marketing, those folks will be very convincing in their belief that you to, can achieve the same success as they have. They will tell you, "You can do it!" This is because they do believe it. Success is a "high" you know this if you've ever experienced it

Many years ago, I heard a man tell an audience, "what the mind can conceive and believe it can achieve" I believe those are true words. However, the obstacle in this statement is **believe**?

You can easily get caught up in someone else's success and envision yourself in similar circumstance. The problem is once left to your own devices the second guessing begins as you face the facts that it's up to you and you alone to make your own success happen.

I can't tell you that you won't be the exception, but, 99% will not execute properly or fail to even begin the process. Therefore, before you invest one penny be sure in your own mind this is a program which will work for you and that your abilities, skill sets and finances support the risk involved.

The next question you need to ask, is this a fad or is it an enduring lifestyle?

AMWAY, founded in 1959 is a Multi-Level Marketing multi-billion-dollar company and has been an institution for over fifty years. It is a Network Marketing company, the people involved in Amway have incorporated this product line into their daily lives. Mary Kay cosmetics is another Multi-Level Marketing multi-billion-dollar company. Avon and Tupperware are also household names built on a direct Network Marketing business model. However, can you picture yourself doing this sales work or can you believe you are one of the few who can achieve success in Network Marketing?

Chapter Three

Richard Kiyosaki, Author of "Rich Dad Poor Dad" and a number of other motivational books endorses Network Marketing even though he admits he has not done it.

He breaks people down into four groups; employees, self-employed, business owners and investors. He is correct in his definition of each group.

Mr. Kiyosaki, places Network Marketing in the business owner group. I agree with this, but, once again I ask you, are you cut out to be a business owner?

The following will make you think about this question and more to the point give you an understanding of all that is involved.

Starting a Business:

Identify your reasons.
1. Being your own boss.
2. Setting your own schedule.
3. Improving your standard of living.
4. Providing a needed product or service.
5. Self-satisfaction.

<u>Do a self-analysis.</u>
1. Are you a leader.
2. Do you like to make your own decisions?
3. Do others turn to you for help.
4. Do you enjoy competition.
5. Do you have will power and self-discipline.
6. Do you plan ahead.
7. Do you like people.
8. Do you get along with all types of people?
9. Are you willing to work 12-14-hour days, weekends and holidays?
10. Do you have the physical stamina to handle the work load?
11. Can you withstand the emotional stress?

12. Are you willing to lower your standard of living to establish your business?
13. Is your family as committed as you are?
14. Are you prepared to invest and possibly lose your investment?
15. Do you have the basic skills necessary to run a successful business?
16. Do you possess the knowledge to grow your business?
17. Do you have a management background?
18. Have you worked at a business similar to the one you want to start?
19. Have you had any formal business training?

20. Are you willing to do the research to learn all the facets of this business?

<u>Feasibility Study</u>
1. Identify and briefly describe the business you plan to start.
2. Identify the product or service you plan to sell.
3. Does this product or service satisfy a need?
4. Will demand exceed supply when competition is factored in.
5. Will you be competitive based on quality, selection, price and service?

<u>Market Analysis.</u>
1. Do you know your customer?
2. Do you understand their needs and wants?

3. Do you know the demographic you are targeting?
4. Are you offering what they want.
5. Will you be a price leader?
6. Will your marketing program be effective?
7. Are you better than your competition?
8. Can you get this across to your customer?

<u>Finances</u>

1. Prepare a personal financial report and determine your net worth?
2. Have you determined how much funding you will require?
3. Have you prepared a realistic budget so that you have staying power?
4. Have you prepared a cash flow analysis?

5. Have you factored in seasonal trends which may affect your business?
6. Do you understand cash flow management?
7. Can you cover personal expenses while the business gets off the ground?
8. Is your family prepared for financial sacrifice if necessary?

<u>Advice</u>

A Business which will not provide you with a complete information package on their offering in order for you to make an informed decision is suspect.

<u>Proceed with caution</u>.

Be absolutely sure your reasoning is sound and that it is confirmed by competent advisors.

I believe if you follow the steps laid out as follows you will have put together the necessary information to make an informed decision on the business your looking to start or acquire.

That being said it should be clear to you now all that's involved in owning a business. The funding needed and the time you must commit to working can be a deal breaker.

A Personal Perspective;
Network marketing is another avenue to explore. One which does not require the huge start-up costs or an end of life as you now know it outcome.

I owned my own store during the early 1980's. There wasn't a worse time to be a

small business owner. I told myself that I
was my own man, but the reality was this,
the store owned me and I was trapped.
After two years I got out, the cost was high,
I walked away broke. In those two years I
had made almost $400,000 but in the end
after the costs and expenses of doing
business I had nothing left.
This was the best learning experience of my
life and the most, costly!

I returned into the workforce and made a
good living until retiring a couple of years
ago. I guess you could say I was lucky.

Today I write books, short stories and post
articles on Linkedin.

I have written this book to tell you, if you
can Sell then Network Marketing may be for

you. If the thought of selling makes you uncomfortable in any way, then walk away.

<u>Do the Work;</u>

<u>Feasibility Study Outline</u>

A feasibility study is an important step in business development. It provides you with a framework and the decision points needed for an analysis in your business development. The outline below can be used to help you through the feasibility study process. However, not all feasibility studies are alike. The elements to include in a feasibility study vary according to the type of the business venture analyzed and the kind of market

opportunities identified.
Below is a listing of typical factors to include.
However, this may not be a complete listing
of the factors that should be considered in
your specific situation.
The success of a feasibility study is based on
the careful identification and assessment of
all of the important issues for a business'
success.
Depending on the business project,
additional items may also be important.
Remember, the basic premise of a feasibility
study is to determine the potential for
success of your proposed business venture.

Description of the Project:
Identification and exploration of business

scenarios:

- Identify alternative scenarios or business models of what the project will entail, how it will be organized, and how it will generate profits. These may come from the idea assessment or market assessment that you may have already completed.
- Eliminate scenarios that don't make sense.
- Flesh-out the scenario(s) that appear to have potential for further exploration.

Define the project and alternative scenarios:

- Describe the type and quality of product(s) or service(s) to be marketed.

- Outline the general business model (i.e. how the business will make money).
- Include the technical processes including size, location, kind of inputs, etc.
- Specify the time horizon from the time the project is initiated until it is up and running at capacity.

Relationship to the surrounding geographical area:

- Outline the economic and social impact on local communities. Describe the environmental impact on the surrounding area.

Market Feasibility:

- This can be based on a market assessment that you may have already completed (i.e. Demographics).

Industry description:

- Describe the size and scope of the industry, market and/or market segment(s).
- Estimate the future direction of the industry, market and/or market segment(s).
- Describe the nature of the industry, market and/or market segment(s). Is it stable or going through rapid change and restructuring?
- Identify the life-cycle of the industry, market and/or market segment(s). Is

it emerging, growing, mature, or declining?

Industry competitiveness:

- Describe the industry concentration. Are there just a few large producers or many small producers?
- Describe the major competitors? Will you compete directly against them?
- Analyze the barriers to entry of new competitors into the market or industry. Can new competitors enter easily?
- Analyze the concentration and competitiveness of input suppliers and product/service/ buyers.
- Describe the price competitiveness of your product/service.

Market potential:

- Identify whether the product will be sold into a commodity market or a differentiated product/service market.
- Identify the demand and usage trends of the market or market segment in which the product or service will participate.
- Examine the potential for emerging, niche or segmented market opportunities.
- Explore the opportunity and potential for a branded product.
- Assess market usage and your potential share of the market or market segment.

Access to market outlets:

- Identify the potential buyers of the product/service and the associated marketing costs.
- Investigate the product/service distribution system and the costs involved.

Sales projection:

- Estimate sales.
- Carefully identify and assess the accuracy of the underlying assumptions in the sales projection.
- Project sales under various assumptions (i.e. selling prices, services provided, etc.).

Technical Feasibility

Facility needs:

- Estimate the size and type of facilities required.
- Investigate the need for related receiving areas, equipment, etc.

Suitability of production technology:

- Investigate and compare technology providers.
- Determine reliability and competitiveness of technology (proven or unproven, state-of-the-art, etc.).
- Identify limitations or constraints of the technology.

Availability and suitability of site
Investigate access to:

- receiving

- parking
- access/egress
- labor
- utility inputs (electricity, natural gas, water, etc.)
- Investigate potential emissions problems.
- Analyze other environmental impacts.
- Identify regulatory requirements.
- Explore economic development incentives.

Procurement:
- Estimate the amount of inventory needed
- Investigate the current and future

availability and access to suppliers.
- Assess the quality and cost from suppliers.

Other inputs:
- Investigate the availability of labor including wage rates, skill level, etc.
- Assess the potential to access and attract qualified management personnel.

Financial/Economic Feasibility

Estimate the total capital requirements:
- Assess the "seed capital" needs of the business project during the investigation process and start-up, and how these needs will be met.

- Estimate capital requirements for facilities, equipment and inventories.
- Estimate working capital needs.
- Estimate start-up capital needs until revenues are realized at full capacity.
- Estimate contingency capital needs due to construction delays, technology malfunction, market access delays, etc.
- Estimate other capital needs.

Estimate equity and credit needs:
- Estimate equity needs.
- Identify alternative equity sources and capital availability - family, SBA, local investors, angle investors, venture capitalists, etc.

- Estimate credit needs.
- Identify and assess alternative credit sources - banks, government (i.e. direct loans or loan guarantees), grants and local and state economic development incentives.

Business Plan:

Budget expected costs and returns of various alternatives:

- Estimate the expected revenue, costs, profit margin and expected net profit.
- Estimate the sales needed to break-even.
- Estimate the returns under various, price and sales levels. This may involve identifying "best case", "typical", and "worst case" scenarios.

- Assess the reliability of the underlying assumptions of the analysis (prices, efficiencies, market access, market penetration, etc.)
- Benchmark against industry averages and/or competitors (cost, margin, profits, ROI, etc.).
- Identify limitations or constraints of the economic analysis.
- Calculate expected cash flows during the start-up period and when the business reaches capacity.
- Prepare pro forma income statement, balance sheet, and other statements of when the business is fully operating.

Business Plan Outline:
Contact Information:

This document contains confidential information. It is disclosed to you for informational purposes only. Its contents shall remain the property of and shall be returned to when requested. This is a business plan and does not imply an offering of securities.

Contents:

Executive Summary

1. Business Opportunity
2. Product/Service Description
3. Current Business Position
4. Financial Potential
5. The Request

NETWORK MARKETING

Company Background

1. Business Description
2. Company History
3. Current Position and Business Objectives
4. Ownership

Products

1. Product Overview
2. Competitive Analysis
3. Suppliers and Inventory
4. Research and Development

Services

1. Service Descriptions
2. Competitive Comparison
3. Service Delivery
4. Research and Development

The Industry, Competition and Market

1. Industry Definition

2. Primary Competitors
3. Market Size
4. Market Growth
5. Customer Profile

Marketing Plan

1. Competitive Advantage
2. Pricing
3. Distribution Channels
4. Promotional Plan
5. Feedback

Operating Plan

1. Location
2. Facility
3. Operating-Equipment
4. Suppliers and Vendors
5. Personnel Plan
6. General Operations

Management, Organization and Ownership

1. Management/Principals
2. Organizational Structure

The undersigned ("Recipient") hereby agrees that all financial and other information ("Information") that it has and will receive is confidential and will not be disclosed to any individual or entity without prior written consent.
The Information shall remain the property of and shall be returned to promptly at its request together with all copies made thereof.

Recipient acknowledges that no remedy of law may be adequate to compensate for a violation of this Agreement and Recipient hereby agrees that in addition to any legal or other rights that may be available in the event of a breach hereunder, may seek equitable relief to enforce this Agreement in any Court of competent jurisdiction.

NETWORK MARKETING

Date   Signature

This is a business plan and does not imply
an offering of securities.

Organizational/Managerial Feasibility
Business structure:
- Identify the proposed legal structure
  of the business.
- Outline the staffing and governance
  structure of the business along with
  lines of authority and decision-
  making structure.
- Identify any potential joint venture
  partners, alliances or other important
  stakeholders.
- Identify the availability of skilled and

experienced business managers.
- Identify the availability of consultants and service providers with the skills needed to realize the project, including legal, accounting, industry experts, etc.

Business founders:
- Character matters - are the people involved of outstanding character?
- Do the founders have the "fire in the belly" required to take the project to completion?
- Do the founders have the skills and ability to complete the project?
- What key individuals will lead the project?
- Is there a reward system for the

founders? Is it based on business performance?

- Have the founders organized other successful businesses?

Study Conclusions:

- Identify and describe alternative business scenarios and models.
- Compare and contrast scenarios based on goals of the group.
- Outline criteria for decision making among alternatives.

Your Next Step;

After the feasibility study has been completed and presented to the leaders of the project, they should carefully study and analyze the conclusions and underlying assumptions. Next, the leaders will be faced with deciding which course of action to pursue.

Potential courses of action include:

- Choosing the most viable business scenario or model, finalizing the business plan and proceeding with creating and operating the business.
- Identifying additional scenarios for further study.

OR

- Deciding that a viable business opportunity is not available and moving to end the business investigation process.
- Following another course of action.

Due Diligence

<u>Key Questions to Answer:</u>

1. Are the financial statements that you have received accurate?
2. Is the Inventory in "Good and Re-saleable" condition?
3. What is the condition and value of the Assets?
4. How effective and committed are the employees?
5. What is the overall picture of industry and the competition?
6. What has the company done to market itself?
7. How strong is the sales team?
8. Will the company's contracts continue under your ownership?

9. What can you do to increase the Revenues and Profits?
10. Based upon what you learn, does the business have a viable future?
11. Does the business meet the criteria of The Ten Commandments?
12. Is this a "Good" business?

<u>Categories to Cover:</u>

1. Financials
2. Assets
3. Sales
4. Marketing
5. Employees
6. Systems
7. Competition
8. Customers
9. Contracts
10. Suppliers

11. Legal and Corporate

<u>Things to Do Before Official Start Date</u>

- Get all Materials required prior to start date
- Advise Seller in writing of official start date and copy to attorney
- Advise accountant of projected start date and confirm their availability
- Confirm project fee from accountant
- Meet with accountant and review the to do lists and targeted completion dates
- Compile a list of everything that needs investigating, note the person responsible and set target completion dates
- Break the tasks down by department (sales, accounting,

employees, assets, etc.). Keep a separate list for each. As each task is completed, cross it off the list.

- Confirm hours that business will be open and available for your work
- Confirm the area where you can work and have some privacy
- Scout the area for a local café or other meeting place
- Arrange with seller to meet all employees and confirm your accessibility to everything
- Arrange to meet with each employee prior to starting and advise your requirements
- Have the seller advise you the point person for your specific and individual information and inquiries
- Begin to set up meetings with all key suppliers and customers

- Outline what work must be done on premises and what can be done when you don't have access to the business (i.e. shopping the competition).

<u>Key Points to Remember:</u>

- Keep the "to do" list current.
- Monitor to do lists daily for everyone
- Schedule all of the tasks to be covered in less time than you have to complete the DD. Leave extra time to revisit certain areas
- Take all your documents home each evening
- Keep a separate listing for all of the "things to do" after the purchase.

Whenever an idea crosses your mind write it down.
- Keep index cards on you and note everything that comes across your mind

FINANCIALS
1. Income Statement

<u>Need to Know:</u>

- Do the financial statements have adequate backup?
- Are the costs correct?
- Has anything been hidden?
- Have the financial statements been properly prepared?
- Is there any questionable accounting?

- Are the financial statements a true reflection of the health of the business?
- What has been the growth rate of the different categories that comprise Revenues?
- What Expenses, if any, can be reduced or must be increased?
- Have there been any "extraordinary" items or one-time occurrences
- Any legal or professional fees that don't seem in line. This may indicate a pending lawsuit or work that may have had to be done for an IRS audit

Supporting Documentation:

1. The company's Income Statements going back as far as possible. Or if

you have access you only need the last five.
2. Company tax returns going back as far as possible but a minimum of 3 years
3. Comparative report outlining all Revenue and Expense items from one year to the next. If necessary, the accountant can use the statements and put together a spreadsheet with this information that will allow you to perform individual comparisons (i.e. in Advertising costs) from one year to the next.
4. Projected operating financing statements if any available from the Seller.
5. Projected Revenue and Expense statements that you must do

6. The chart of accounts (a listing of each different item in the financial statements)

2. The Balance Sheet

(a) Accounts Receivable

<u>Need to Know:</u>

- Trace client invoices to see how long it takes them to pay. Track down each invoice to see how many days after invoicing was their payment received.
- How does each client pay? Check? Cash? Credit card?
- Can the check payers be converted to credit card payments?

- Verify the amounts owing against the customer's records. This can be done easily by calling random accounts.
- Any Receivables due from employees? If so, ask them about this.
- Compare the AR over the past years. Any trends?
- What are the company's general terms of sale and is it comparable to the competition?
- Do the customers respect the terms?
- Do any clients get special year-end allowances, volume rebates or any other "bonus" that must be accounted for? Remember to reduce the amount of the purchase by what the customer will be getting for

sales that were generated in the current year which you will not be receiving any credit.

- Which employee is responsible for the credit? Is it a full-time position? What are their challenges? What are their suggestions for improvement?

Required:

1. Reports outlining the amounts due from all customers, employees or any other party.
2. Aged Trial Balances of each receivable listed in #1
3. Copies of customer invoices, company deposit books and bank statements
4. The Balance Sheet going back several fiscal periods.

(b) Inventory

<u>Need to Know:</u>

- How much is "Good and Re-saleable" *(those items in which the quantities on hand represent the amounts which have been sold in the previous 12 months).*
- Inventory accuracy

Required:

1. Inventory Report by item
2. Sales report by item for the past 12 months
3. Inventory Counting Company?
4. Hire individual to help count audit the counting process

(c) Furniture and Equipment

<u>Need to Know:</u>

- Is the equipment working?
- How long can you expect it to produce Revenue?
- What are maintenance costs?
- Have the manufacturers send in a service rep to evaluate it?
- Determine the major breakdowns you can expect
- What warrantees are still in place?
- What work/maintenance was done on the equipment in the past year?
- What are replacement costs?
- Can you afford to replace these if required?

- Which items are owned, which are leased?
- Do the Leasing Companies offer trade in allowances?
- Remember what was discussed regarding computers and office equipment

Required:

1. Listing of all items
2. Valuation report
3. Depreciation schedule indicating accumulated and remaining
4. Lease contracts
5. Maintenance contracts
6. Listing of all equipment manufacturers

(d) Liabilities

<u>Need to Know:</u>

- Verify the supplier statements with the company's records.
- Have each supplier send you an updated statement
- Any obligations that you will assume must have reconciliation and explanation from the party to whom you will have the obligation.

<u>Required:</u>

1. Accounts Payable listing
2. Supplier statements

3. Letter/Documentation from all parties to whom you will be obligated financially

PRO FORMA STATEMENTS

<u>Things to Remember:</u>

- Be extremely conservative and use a formula that will clearly dictate the downside.
- Don't "fall in love with the business" before you own it.
- You want to know the worst-case scenario.
- Include the added debt
- Included a provision for your salary
- Take the cost of professional fees and add 20%,

- Allow for a decrease in sales in the first year of 10, 15 and 20%.
- Include a provision for unexpected major expenses in case of equipment replacement.
- Allow for the seasonality of the business (do the Pro Forma on a month-by-month basis beginning with the month in which you may realistically take over the business).
- Take all of these so-called negatives and work them every which way into the Pro Forma Income Statement to determine what the business will look like.
- Do not make the mistake of playing with the numbers until they look good. Play with them so you can digest how you will be able to deal with them should they turn bad.

- Learn what your monthly break-even point will be.
- You want to know how much you have to generate each month in sales so that the Gross Margins cover your Fixed Expenses.

Required:

1. Prepare an Excel Spreadsheet with all of the various categories and the "play around" with the numbers.

BANKING
<u>Need to Know:</u>

- Review all bank statements
- Examine any Loan/Line of Credit accounts. Any trends from year to

year? Any seasonality meaning does the business use the line more at a specific time of year (perhaps in slower seasons)?
- What Interest rates are being paid"
- Any loans that are not guaranteed by the Seller that can be assigned to you once you purchase the business?
- Who signs the company checks?

Supporting Documentation:

1. Copies of all bank statements for the past 3 years
2. Documentation on any existing loans
3. Listing of all company bank accounts, numbers, institution and signees.

SALES
<u>Need to Know:</u>

- What do the salespeople do on a typical day?
- How are company's products 'pitched' to customers? Have each salesperson do a sales presentation for you
- How are new customers solicited?
- Who are the top salespeople?
- How long have they been with the company?
- Will they stay?
- What happens if they leave?
- What are the company's sales policies?
- Are the policies organized?

- Does every customer have a different deal?
- What latitude does a salesperson have with the clients?
- How long are clients retained?
- Are the company's products a one-time sale?
- Are there repeat orders?
- What percentage of the company's business comes from repeat sales?
- What is the cost to obtain a new customer?
- Are the sales done in house?
- Do the salesman do any traveling?
- Are the clients local, national, international?
- Are there any remote salespeople?
- Do the salespeople report to the office each day?

- Are they salaried or commission based?
- What is their total benefits package?
- Is it within industry standards?
- Who does the sales forecasts and budgets?
- Are the budgets monitored daily, weekly, monthly?
- What happens if sales fall below budget?
- Is there a sales manager? What is his/her role? Who do they report to?
- Do the salespeople seem to like the manager?
- What training does the company provide for new salespeople?
- What training is done on an ongoing basis?

- How difficult is it to recruit new salespeople?
- How many orders are called in each day?
- Do the sales have to be chased down?
- Are orders lost or gained based upon price?
- What are the salespeople's biggest challenges?
- What recommendations do the salespeople have for increasing Revenues?
- What is the entire sales procedure from solicitation to closing and shipping?
- What systems are in place for follow up? Is this a manual system? Does each salesperson have their own

"way" of doing things or is there a standard sales system in place?

- What role does technology play in the sales function?
- How automated is the sales department?
- What costs are involved to fully automate the sales process?
- Could a system be put into place? Has the company previously considered this and what information can you get that will show what was previously done?
- How open are the sales people to change?

Supporting Documentation:

1. List of top customers that contribute at least 75% of total sales

2. List of each salespersons top five accounts broken down by sales with sales terms and commentary
3. Sales policies
4. Discount/pricing structure
5. Sales staff to provide suggestions in list form of what can be done to increase the business
6. Sales Report by salesperson and what has been their performance to date

MARKETING
<u>Need to Know:</u>

- Does the company have a Marketing Plan?
- Have they followed it?
- What has been successful?
- What has failed?

- What were the costs of each campaign?
- Does the company have a clear definition of what business they are in?
- Does the company really know who their customer is?
- How focused is the company on marketing their products or services to the right potential customers?
- What methods are used to sell more products to the current client base?
- Does the company spend more effort on getting new customers or on increasing their volume with current clients?
- How much money does the company spend on marketing each year?

- Does the company know why their customers buy from them?
- Is the company clear on what its strengths and weaknesses are?
- Are the company's strengths made clear to the customers?
- If the customers were asked to list the company's strengths and weaknesses would these be the same as the company's list?
- Is the company focused on delivering the message of its strengths and improving upon its weaknesses?
- Does the company make it a priority to continually test new marketing ideas?
- Are new marketing programs analyzed in detail to really

understand what is and isn't working?

- When the company finds a strategy that "seems" to be working, do they stick with it or do they keep trying to improve upon it?
- Ask each employee what is the single biggest unique thing that the company offers potential customers
- Ask the customers the same question.
- Ask each employee what is the most important factor that determines whether a customer buys from them or the competition.
- Ask the same thing to the customers.
- Are the salespeople selling the same benefits that the marketing team is preaching?

<u>Supporting Documentation:</u>

1. Copy of current Marketing Plan if available
2. Detailed commentary on the Marketing Plan results of each campaign, costs, business generated, etc.
3. Copy of all company marketing materials
4. Report from sales/marketing employees on marketing activity and suggestions for the future

EMPLOYEES
<u>Need to Know:</u>

- What is the job description, compensation plans and years of service of each employee?
- Have any employees been promised any compensation increases or other benefits?
- Any labor disputes?
- Have any employees indicated their desire to leave the company after the purchase?
- What fears and concerns do the employees have about your pending purchase?
- Do the employees seem favorable to the purchase?
- Identify the "key" employees
- Has the competition recently hired any of the company's employees?
- Has the business hired any of the competitor's employees?

- Do they seem genuinely interested in helping you build the business?
- Do any mention that they believe the business has a lot of opportunity?
- What are your initial impressions of each employee?
- How helpful and knowledgeable are they about the questions you ask them?
- Does there seem to be any "cliques" within the company?
- What evidence do you sense of any office politics?

Supporting Documentation:

1. Organizational Chart outlining who reports to whom?

2. Job Description, Compensation (itemized salary, bonus, non-financial compensation such as car allowance, expense account, etc.), years of service, SSN for each employee with commentary regarding any promises made by the Seller to any of them
3. Copies of any Employee Agreements
4. Copies of any Consulting Agreements
5. Employee files with memos for reprimands or any other disciplinary action or warning
6. Listing of any labor disputes, work stoppages, union certifications (pending, considered or otherwise)
7. Copy of Employee Benefit Program (medical, retirement)

8. Summary of company incentive plans, including profit sharing
9. Confidentiality Agreements if any

OPERATING SYSTEMS

- Whatever systems are in place have them evaluated.
- how does the business operate and what role does technology/systems play in making these operations flow quicker and more effectively?
- The business' ability to produce accurate and useful reports is a direct indication of the business' overall level of organization.
- Does the company produce reports that provide financial, sales,

inventory analysis on a monthly basis?

- Ask everyone, including the Seller, what reports they use and review them.
- Ask each employee which reports they would like to see on a monthly basis.
- Get a copy of the software manuals. Locate their website and call the company. Have them give you the name of a local dealer. Call the dealer, explain what you are doing and arrange to meet with them. While avoiding techno talk, have them explain what the system can do for you.
- If the business is not using any systems for sales or operations you must determine what the costs will

be to get these systems in place.
They are usually not expensive but
there is a cost

- Contact the industry associations
  and determine if there is any
  software that is available that is
  specific to the industry (most have
  them).
- Does the company have a website?
- Who maintains it?
- How much business is done through
  it?
- Do the employees use email?
- Do each of the employees have PCs
  and Internet access?
- If they did, would it help?
- If they do, are they using it and for
  what purposes?
- Is there an employee in charge of
  the systems?

- Does the company outsource for computer maintenance? If so, whom do they use? Arrange to meet with this person and get their input. Usually, these individuals can be a wealth of information once you tell them to speak your language and not in "code" as they tend to do.
- If you have to purchase new systems what will they cost?
- Any lease agreements in place for computer equipment?
- Any contractual obligations for computer maintenance?

Supporting Documentation:

1. Contracts for any equipment leases, maintenance contracts
2. Software manuals

3. Website access, pass code (when purchase completed)
4. Copies of all reports currently being produced

COMPETITION

- Have each salesperson and marketing employee put together the competitive information they have. See what each one has on their own.
- Have the salespeople provide you with a competitive analysis including strengths and weaknesses of each of the competitors and what they believe must be done to beat them.
- Put together a listing of the leading competitors
- Get their price lists, catalogs, etc.

- Visit the different websites
- What do they use as their "hook" to get customers?
- What advertising do they do?
- How many of your clients buy from them as well?
- Do they sell based on price, service, availability, selection?
- Who are the owners?
- Are they bigger than you?
- How long have they been in business?
- Number of employees?
- Obtain a credit rating on them
- On what basis does each one competes with the business?
- What do they seem to do better?
- Is their customer base the same or does it differ? How?

NETWORK MARKETING

Supporting Documentation:

1. All competitive materials available
2. Listing of all major competitors, phone numbers and website address, profiles

CUSTOMERS

<u>Need to Know:</u>

- Meeting them may be difficult
- Consult course for specific strategy
- Try to ascertain if the large accounts appear to be happy with the company
- You must meet with the larger accounts and confirm their ongoing business

<u>Supporting Documentation:</u>

1. See Sales category
2. Report with sales by customer for current year and previous year

CONTRACTS

<u>Supporting Documentation FOR ALL CONTRACTS:</u>

1. Copies of all contracts in each category
2. Do a spreadsheet listing all contracts, terms, expiry date, follow up to be done

(e)Leases

<u>Need to Know:</u>

- What is the lease term?
- Is it transferable?
- What are the renewal options?
- What are the actual costs?
- What's included? Excluded?
- Is the rent current?
- Can you negotiate a new lease as previously outlined (1 or 2 years w/5-year renewal options)?
- If the business relies on other tenants or other nearby businesses for traffic (i.e. a retail location) are they committed long-term to their locations? Get this in writing if you can from the landlord. Does the landlord own other property and where?
- Check out the landlord's reputation with other tenants.

- Ask the employees if they are aware of any problems with the premises (leaks, broken AC, etc.)
- Does the landlord respond quickly to problems?
- Do they have their own "handyman"?

(f) Insurance Policies

<u>Need to Know:</u>

- Are they transferable?
- Do you need them?
- What are the costs to replace the non-transferable but required ones?
- Check out any customer or supplier contracts as they may require that you carry a minimum amount of liability insurance.

- There may be certain laws that are specific to your products/services where insurance policies must be of a certain type and coverage amount. Check this out.

(g) Customer Contracts

<u>Need to Know:</u>

- Are you obligated to respect certain prices, terms, conditions, delivery guarantees, etc. with certain accounts?

(h) Supplier Contracts

<u>Need to Know:</u>

- Are the contracts assignable to a new owner?
- Remember the difference between assignable and transferable
- Is there a transfer fee?
- Do the licensing and distribution rights end if ownership changes?
- How easy will it be for you to renew these contracts when they expire?
- If you cannot keep these contracts how viable is the business?
- Does the licensed merchandise itself act as an anchor to get the customers to buy the generic merchandise?
- What percentage of the business is attributable to these suppliers?
- What are the consequences if the relationship is terminated

immediately? What about in 6 or 12 months?
- Review the course section again as there are many potential hazards with suppliers that need to be reviewed

LEGAL AND CORPORATE

<u>Need to Know:</u> (Have your lawyer participate in this area)

- You want to know what if any, legal issues are pending or may be arise.
- Have the business itself verified from a legal standpoint to be sure that it is an active corporation
- Need a listing of all shareholders and directors

- Be sure all filing fees, licenses, are current.

Supporting Documentation:

1. Copy of company minute books
2. Incorporation documents
3. Copies of all documents related to any ongoing or potential legal proceeding

<u>Summary</u>

- Begin to gather information the moment a business becomes of interest to you.
- Be sure you identify the precise business category.
- Do your homework.
- Work quickly.

- Get as many resources as possible from the business owner.
- There are tons of resources available to you, but you have to go after them.
- Evaluate everything, because you never know where it can lead.
- Don't be afraid to contact these resources and ask questions, lots of them.
- Be creative in your approach. (You can be anybody you want!)
- Play the role of "hunter" and information is your "prey."
- Salespeople love to talk, so speak to them whenever possible.
- Take detailed notes and, when going "undercover," remember to note your story in case you want to call some of these people back.

- Establish a clear set of questions that you want answers on and focus on getting those answers.

Back to Network Marketing:

Why have I included the too do list for investigating a mainstream business start-up, purchase, or acquisition? What does this have to do with Network Marketing?

1. Business is business regardless of what kind of business it is.
2. Shortcuts or reckless disregard for establishing the facts equal failure!
3. Understanding the facts is mandatory.
4. Going into a new venture prepared gives you a fighting chance to succeed.

5. Your able to present a credible defense to your naysayers.
6. You know what you're getting yourself into!

Chapter Four

Now, to explore the positive and negative aspects of this Network Marketing opportunity.

Why did I join this Network Marketing company? As I stated previously, first and foremost, I use these products! Secondly, not only do I use this product, I receive pre-IPO shares which will convert to stock when this company goes public. Thirdly, it was an opportunity to get inside to research this company for the book you are now reading.

I have been using a number of these products for a number of weeks now and I am confident and convinced that this product will maintain or improve my good health.

When the company goes public and it takes off like Amazon so much the better. Why do I think this is possible? Because as I stated earlier the folks behind this company are rich and they wouldn't be in this if they didn't believe it will make them even richer. Taking the company public will be very lucrative for those already invested in the company.

The company is "PURE"
(www.livepure.com)

They offer a health & wellness line of products which have been growing in usage across the countries they do business in.

What is most impressive is that five of these products are listed and recommended in the PDR, (Physician's Desk Reference) this is the prescribers manual for medical professionals.

They are, Health Trim Cleanse (Liquid), Daily Build, Grape Energy, Cacao 360 Complete Shake and Metabolic One.

I want to address the 7 Day Detox! You can do the detox for 7 days or 28 days.

People have been detoxing for better health for many years, but the side benefit with this cleanse is that you lose weight with this program as well.

If you need to lose some weight, this is the plan for you.

You can do it for 7 days and then skip 28 days and do it again. Or, if you are a couple, you both can do it for 14 days. Some people have balked saying this is expensive, but how much do you spend on groceries? How much of what you purchase is adding to your health problems? Believe me, I have used this cleanse and after the first few days I felt a significant change.

Who couldn't stand to lose a few pounds while removing the toxins from your body? Here is the introduction to the plan. A comprehensive PDF is available as an easy to follow guide.

7-Day PURE Detox / Metabolic Reset

"We live in a toxic world and our bodies are bombarded with chemicals and other potentially harmful substances on a regular basis. These environmental toxins are often in the food we eat, the water we drink, and the air we breathe. They are also found in most of the commercial products we use daily. Our bodies are designed to deal with and eliminate these toxic substances; however, we can become encumbered by them, which puts a heavy burden on our innate systems of elimination. Ultimately, over time these toxins take a toll on our health leading to low energy levels, extra body weight, and feelings of malaise and brain fog.

The average person also consumes far too much processed foods and added sugar. Sugar is hidden in places you would least expect it. The average American consumes an estimated 77 to 88 pounds of sugar every year. This is the equivalent of nearly 5 ½ full size candy bars every single day. Most people do not realize most packaged and processed foods contain added sugar. It is doubtful the typical person would lay out 5 to 6 full size candy bars every day and say to themselves, "I'm going to eat these and not worry about their impact on my health." Yet, most of us consume this much sugar every single day. Over 90% of the sugar we consume comes from processed and packaged foods and not from candy and desserts. Furthermore, the typical person consumes almost 200 lbs. of refined flour and cereal products annually. Too much sugar and refined carbohydrates contribute to weight gain and poor health.

The 7-Day PURE Detox program was developed to assist your body in ridding itself of these environmental toxins and waste, avoid processed foods, added sugars, and refined flour and to change your focus to eating whole foods. During your 7-Day journey, as you give your body a break from your typical eating patterns, your energy levels will soar, you will find new found mental clarity and focus, and you will likely shed a few extra pounds along the way.

PURE provides a Food Guide to help you prepare a shopping list. A Daily Calendar is provided for your shopping list to better prepare for food quantities to be purchased. Meals are recommended on a Daily Calendar."

There are over thirty-five different products formulated to address living a healthy lifestyle.

Chapter Five

Satisfying customers, PURE, use a multi-channel communication network.
The Baby Boomer Generation, born between 1946 and 1964, accommodated customer needs by brick and mortar store fronts.

Generation X, born between 1965-1979, became a little more demanding. This group no longer expected products to merely cover their needs. Once they knew the benefits and advantages of the product, they expected added value.

X'ers however are caught in the middle of two changing paradigms, old and new.

The now dominate Millennial Generation includes those born between 1980 and 1994. They are the technology-savvy generation, who cannot function without a computer and a I-Phone.

The majority are actively engaged in social media, like Facebook, Twitter, YouTube, Instagram, etc.

The Millennial Generation is much more demanding than its predecessors. The Millennials not only expect the products they purchase to meet their needs and tastes they demand added value and justification by the provider as to its composition.

This now requires the product, brand or company to create an experience that specifically identifies with each individual customer.

The Millennial generation must feel important and expect their contribution to be valued. They must feel they are being heard.

Millennials no longer require the antiquated communication methods of decades past. They live in the now and utilize multi-channel media communication which is relevant to their interests and beliefs.

PURE technologies integrate multi-channel communication with customers and

Independent Business Owners to execute extreme service and product satisfaction.

Millennials, need for health and wellness products fits perfectly with PURE's products. The workplace environments today and tomorrow will see the Millennials changing employment a number of times throughout their career.

The PURE business opportunity is an ideal fit for many of them in their search for accomplishment, recognition and financial independence.

Anyone who has ever been involved in a Network Marketing or Direct Sales company will find as they explore PURE, that it has the potential for a level of personal success in my opinion, if your cut out for this type of business.

One last thing to consider;

The Government wants to rename Social Security payments so the government can claim that all the social security recipients are receiving entitlements thus putting them in the same category as welfare, and food stamp recipients. The Social Security check soon will be referred to as a Federal Benefit Payment?

This is NOT a benefit It is OUR money, paid out of our earned income! Not only did we all contribute to Social Security but our employers did too! It totals 15% of our income before taxes. Social Security, had it been conservatively invested after 40 years of working you'd have more than $1,000,000+ dollars in your account.

This is our personal investment. Upon retirement, if you took out 4% per year, you'd receive $40,000 per year, or $4,000 per month. The highest benefit now paid is $2788 per month and then Part B has to be deducted from your check.

$4,000 is over three times more than today's average Social Security benefit of $1,230 per month, according to the Social Security Administration. Imagine how much better most average-income people could live in retirement if our government had invested our money in low-risk interest-earning accounts.

Instead, the folks in Washington pulled off a bigger "Ponzi scheme" than Bernie Madoff. They took our money and used it elsewhere. Then they "Conveniently forgot "that it was OUR money they were taking which they don't pay interest on.

Recently they've told us that the money won't support us for very much longer. They NEVER say this about welfare payments? Now, they're calling it a "benefit," as if we never worked to earn every penny of it. This is stealing!

I'm sure you've heard the talk on universal basic income, pay everyone the same minimum benefit. What's behind this and what are the ramifications of another questionable boondoggle by our elected officials. Of course, they won't be subject to this as they are not subject to anything "We the People" are held too.

We earned our right to Social Security and Medicare. Demand that our legislators find a way to keep Social Security and Medicare going for the sake of the 92% of our population who need it.

The government mismanaged our money and stole from the system, so that it's now going broke and they have the audacity to call today's seniors "vultures" in an attempt to cover their ineptitude!

The Baby Boomers may feel threatened by this, but, it's unlikely they will see their benefits cut or lost. The ramifications would destroy the country. However, Generation X and the Millennials along with the generations to follow may very well see this become the reality.

The Baby Boomers saw the employer pension go away to be replaced with 401K's. If you do the math, you'll find that this money, your money, is played with by those who have no concern for your financial future. If your lucky you may get the money you put into your 401K and a portion of your employers' contribution back, but, don't bother to look for the returns you were promised they just aren't there!

Market corrections wipe out gains in high return funds. The one's your encouraged to put your money in.

If you need a reason to consider creating another income stream then securing your financial future is the best reason I can think of.

Chapter Six

The following is the communications I've received from my sponsor over the past six months.

If you get into a Network Marketing company, you can expect to receive this type of information and much more.

The purpose is to keep you motivated and engaged. However, what happens when the one sending you these updates becomes disenchanted and grabs on to the next great Network Marketing plan?

As you read on, you'll find out!

Hey Everyone,

I wanted to send out an email to share something that our upline guy came up with. For many of you, there seems to be some confusion or exasperation in getting started in your business.

We all got into this business for 2 reasons: better health and better finances. We all agree that the products are great and second to none, but the financial portion has many perplexed. I will show you his PowerPoint that he is using. First, I want to dispel some myths.

When we got started in this business, I think the prevailing mindset was: I need to go sign up a bunch of people to make this work. That's great, BUT It only takes 2 to get started. YES, it only takes 2. As you will see in his presentation. If you are serious about making your business go, then follow along.

The idea behind this business is "everyone is doing their part". This simply means, you start with the auto ship. THEN you **find 2 (just 2) people** that are serious about this business and get them **going on the products doing auto ship** just like you- AND **they have committed to getting 2.** Not 10 15 or 20 but 2. just 2, only 2. I think you get the, concept.

You help them to get their 2. You actually get on the phone or go with them to help them present PURE. Then it is their job to help their 2 people get 2 each. and so on. So, your minimum commitment is to be on auto ship and get 2 others to do the same.

The question I pose to you, which you will pose to 2 others (and yes, it is fine to get as many as you want) is this, would you spend 129.00 a month (minimum auto ship amount) to make from $250 to $1,000 a month? **It's really this easy.**

Let me say that this line of people 2 by 2 by 2 etc. is dependent on each and every one doing their share, so a commitment needs to be made for each of you to do your part.

The power of multiplication is staggering. I am putting in this chart just so you can visualize 1 penny that is doubled every day

for 30 days. **Day 1:** $.01

Day 2: $.02
Day 3: $.04
Day 4: $.08
Day 5: $.16
Day 6: $.32
Day 7: $.64
Day 8: $1.28
Day 9: $2.56
Day 10: $5.12
Day 11: $10.24
Day 12: $20.48
Day 13: $40.96
Day 14: $81.92

Day 15: $163.84
Day 16: $327.68
Day 17: $655.36
Day 18: $1,310.72
Day 19: $2,621.44
Day 20: $5,242.88
Day 21: $10,485.76
Day 22: $20,971.52
Day 23: $41,943.04
Day 24: $83,886.08
Day 25: $167,772.16
Day 26: $335,544.32
Day 27: $671,088.64
Day 28: $1,342,177.28
Day 29: $2,684,354.56
Day 30: $5,368,709.12

Now take this same concept by getting 2 people
to do auto ship like you and them 2 etc.

NETWORK MARKETING

Do you know 2 people to talk to today who are into Good Health, Fitness or looking to just lose some weight and feel better?

Hey Guys,

A couple of things to share. One, I have been on the 28-day detox for 7 days and have lost 7 pounds and feeling great with no jitters or tiredness.

I played golf yesterday and felt fine with plenty of energy. I noticed there are some Naysayers that will say the weight loss is from water loss. In this detox, you are drinking a lot of water. whatever your weight is (say 200) then you drink 1/2 of your weight in ounces or 100 ounces of water a day. Between drinking the water and swallowing water in mixing the products, there is no water loss here folks!

I have noticed that almond milk, although tastes
like nothing by itself, is great in the 360 shakes.
I use a vanilla almond milk from Walmart
"Walmart brand" which tastes sweeter with
more vanilla taste than the HEB brand.

Mix and blend this with your chocolate or
vanilla 360, add 4 or 5 cubes of ice and this
actually tastes great, like a real shake. Similar
products on the market today are just
tolerable. This is enjoyable.

We all know Rachel Garcia from her videos. I
got to meet and talk with her at the conference
last week and I found a video she made on the
7-day detox. it is a great approach talking about
how we get busy and our bodies get off center
and need a reset, thus the 7-day detox. here is
the video: the video is only 8 minutes long

https://youtu.be/ZZtjtN3bvDQ

Hey guys, I found this video that I had not seen before that explains the company and its product line.

It is only 9 minutes vs Rachel Garcia's that is 23 minutes. This is also commercially done by

the company itself. check it out. I will be using this one for now on to send to people.

https://youtu.be/2_Zx3dB8oPs

Hey everyone,

I wanted to email you guys about a couple of things. I have been on several connect calls with

CK (even did one with Brig Hart) the last couple of days. If you are not aware, the proper way to talk to a prospect on the phone is with a 3-way call.

Simply tell someone that you have a video you would like them to watch and send it to them at a specific time agreed on. Then you tell them that you will call after the video is thru. I have been using Rachel Garcia's video that is about 26 min long. I send it to the person and say I will call you in about 45 minutes, then I call and talk about PURE and if they are interested, I tell them that at PURE we are all about helping each other working as a team. I explain to them that I want to introduce them to one of my business partners, so when they need to make a call for help or have questions they have already been introduced and spoken to this person who has the answers.

This is when I call CK and he tells them a little about himself and why he is in the business.

He will finish his story then hang up and I finish up with them.

NETWORK MARKETING

Sound's scary? if you go to;

http://pureteamglobal.com

There is a video that actually is a roll play on this very thing. Takes the scary out of it.

You know, CK is waiting by the phone with baited breath waiting to take your call and help you guys.

We all got in this business to make some extra money with products which are great and which work.

So, let's talk to some people and get this done. No, doesn't hurt. The statistics are 1 out of 10 will say yes. If you happen to get your first 9 in a row are no before the 1 who says yes, don't give up. A lot of people quit saying " I talked to 4 people who told me no, this does not work". I know better, and my bank account knows better, and all of the people I just saw and talked to at the conference in Frisco, TX know better as well. let's all make a move forward to achieve the financial independence we all desire.

A fortune cookie I opened a short time ago said, "to make it to the top, you have to get off your bottom". That was a wakeup call for me.

I want to share this the other day. She is in my downline team.

Rose sent me a text that is worth telling everyone about. she said" I have been drinking earthwater and fusion and goyin, daily build, and sulfur, and finally my severe back pain into the SI joint let go!

She said: "You will never know how excited I am".

She goes on to say that she is going to rethink her hip replacement surgery now. That will preach!

So happy for you Rose and glad you are better.

Team, we have some great products with some great testimonies out there use these to grow your business.

As a PA, I am constantly reading material and take continuing medical education. This keeps me up and current on all the latest trends, and treatments etc.

Surround yourself with people that are already doing what you want to be doing. They are trying to instruct and show you how to succeed.

 Our job is to pay attention and do as they say and do!

That's all for now,

NETWORK MARKETING

P.S.

I am doing now what most people won't so I can do what most people can't which is take control of my life.

Now, no excuse, LOL

Hey Guys,

A quick email to give you a little info. I have been asked about our products and some will say, I don't want you to tell me about it until I have taken them for myself to see if they are ok. Or, I have been asked by others, what if someone asks what's in the product?

For both of these questions let me address them together. First of all, as you all know I am a PA and have been practicing for 22 years and I was a Paramedic for 15 years in Dallas before finishing medical school. In my practicing years I do not recall anyone saying, "ok you say I have a sinus infection and you are giving me this and this, what is in that medication?" Or I can't recall anyone asking what is in that IV your squirting in my arm during the middle of their heart attack. People go to the Doctor or Hospital and rarely question the professionals attending to their crisis.

Medications have a long history of doing well for a specific problem and patients use it for that problem and get good results. Which brings me to the PDR. **The Physician's Desk Reference**. This is the "Bible" for prescribers. We medical practitioners use this to tell us what medications are used for what problems, including the side effects and conflicting effects with other medications etc.

So, it is very impressive to me that **5 of our products are in the PDR**. That, in my mind takes away any doubts about their safety, or their legitimacy.

Obviously, each individual needs to evaluate their own particular health situation and talk to their Doctor if needed before starting anything new. But in my mind, these are all plant based "whole food" supplements that are not genetically altered in the lab which can have many great benefits that I think we all are seeing from our personal use. Truth is in the pudding (or in this case the PDR)

Hey guys,

Well Thanksgiving is over and Christmas is coming. Do you realize that in about 6 weeks we will see one of the largest opportunities of the year for our business? That's right, New Year's resolution time. There is a huge uptake in health club memberships, as well as diet, wellness and fitness products sold at this time.

NETWORK MARKETING

So NOW is the time to start laying your foundation for this focus. Not waiting until then when people have already decided on something else. We have great products and all of you who have done the detox program know firsthand how help's you lose weight and feel great.

I have a video that I watched that is really for people who do marketing on the internet, thru Facebook etc. But the points are the same as if you were talking to your neighbor, or your friend about a new product.

Watch the video and I think a lightbulb will go on and you will discover very quickly that we all, me included have approached or prospected or whatever you want to call it - the wrong way! Gone are the days of 'this is great, you need it, buy it now". That doesn't work much anymore. the video is only 16 minutes, so watch and get the AHH Ha moment that I did! Let's get to work and make some money!

https://youtu.be/JnaLUGCoXUl

Hey Guys,

OK, so you have talked to several people and you gotten some interest, but you have also gotten lots of not now, don't have the time, don't have the money, bla bla bla.

Well I think you all have seen CK's great presentation on you and 2. I know that he has talked to many of you about this. I know he will get a copy of this email and if any one of you needs to see it again, or talk to CK more about it, he would be happy to. I will leave his email below for yawl.

I have a script here that I am going to put in for you to say, or email to those that you have talked to in the past and for whatever reason, they were not interested.

With the "you and 2 presentation," this presentation puts a whole new light on things. If you can show a person how they can make 250 to 1000 a month or more thru this simple process then you can convince them in using the "you and 2," their response will be quite different.

Remember "hey I have these great products and you can make some extra money with it, are you interested?" may not work.

Here is my script:

Hi Sally,

I'm from Georgetown, Texas.

I'm just getting back to you with information you requested a while back in regards to making money from home on the Internet.

Are you still looking for a new way to make money from home?

Response

Great, so how long have you been looking for a new business to make money with?

Response

Why are you looking for a business?

Response

How will a home business change your life?

Response

What do you do now for income?

Response

How long have you been doing it? And Do you like it?

Response

Is your job something you can see yourself doing 5-10 years from now?

Response

What type of income are you looking to generate from a home business?

Response

How much time are you able to devote to a start-up business right now?

Response

So, if I can show you that you can make X
amount of dollars, working X hours per week, so
you can make X, which you just told me is very
important to you, do you want to learn how to
do this right away?

Response

Great, you sound like someone I might be able
to help in achieving your goals like I have helped
many other people in similar circumstances
much like yours.

When would be a good time for us to talk in
more detail and discuss how to get you started?

Response

Just like that. Try it.

NETWORK MARKETING

I have been working double duty at the urgent care since the other provider is out on maternity leave, I picked up a lot of her shifts. Working 24 days this month. Leaves little time to send emails etc. But, be for sure that I am working behind the scenes at moving forward in my PURE business.

A couple of things to note:

1. New Years is 1 week away. That means that everyone is going to want to make a new resolution to lose weight and you and I have the answer.

2. I have had allergies for years. For the last 5 years I have lived in Georgetown (Austin) and the allergies are the worst here. We have cedar trees here that bloom and it is soooo bad that the word CEDAR FEVER was coined. Everyone including me has cedar fever with terrible allergies.

BUT, for the first time ever, I do not have any allergies this year. Every year before this one I would take Mucinex, Flonase, Zyrtec, Sudafed and Antihistamine eye drops several times a day. And taking all 5 of those I would barely get by. I have not taken one of any of those this year. Instead, I take Mangosteen, GoYin, and organic Sulfur. These 3 products are life savers. no runny nose, no itchy watery eyes, no constant nagging cough and no nasal drainage and congestion at night. You guys around the Austin area (or any area where allergies are a problem) spread the word that you know a better way!

Another thing I would like to mention is marketing your business. I have been doing ALOT of studying on how to market a business whether it be online or in person. The fact is, most of us go about marketing all wrong. People want to buy, but do not want to be sold. Most of us start to tell someone about our

company or opportunity and we blast them
with things such as: we have a great
daily vitamin that has 40 minerals and vitamins
and you need it. We have a great detox
program and you need it. When someone hears
that, unless they are your child, husband, wife,
or parent, then their shields go up. People do
not want to be told what they need. Every
person has "Pain Points" in their life. It could be
a weight issue, a pain issue, an indigestion
issue, an anxiety issue, a need to make more
income issue, and on and on. We are all looking
for an answer to our "pain issue".

The way to properly approach the subject with
someone is to first listen. Listen to what their
issues are. In medical school 25 years ago, they
taught us that if you listen to your patient long
enough, they would tell you what is wrong. It is
very true. The same thing goes for your
prospect. If you listen to them, they will tell you
what is going on with them in their life.

Maybe they are tight on finances and would like extra income. Maybe they would love the time freedom of staying home with the kids rather than working every day. maybe they have back pain that nags at them daily. Perhaps some indigestion issues that cannot be figured out.

Once you find their pain point, then you can discuss with them how you have an answer for them. A proven way to make their problem better. Although we do not claim any cures, we have mounds of testimonies that are proof that these products can be a great answer to a need (or pain point).

You don't have to look very hard to find many testimonials on the PURE products. There are testimonials that range from making money, to helping with chronic pain, helping with indigestion, with sleep problems, with weight loss, and on and on and on. The point is, we have a great company. We have a great compensation plan. We have great products. We have great testimonials. All of this adds up to being able to approach someone, listen to their "pain points" in life, and offer a solution to their problem. Blasting them with your opportunity up front does not work in most cases. Maybe someone already takes a great vitamin and does not want to change. Maybe someone already takes a great sleep aid and does not want to change. If you lead the conversation and do not listen first about what your customer needs, then you could lose out on a potential sale and new partner.

We offer so many different options in our company. Some people might be looking for a great workout supplement. I would suggest that most of the older PURE IBOs do not talk much if any to prospects upfront about the workout products. Working out and getting the best nutrition, energy and rebuilding of muscle and tissue is not an interest to you as the presenter, but may be exactly what their pain point is. Until you have a conversation and listen to them, you will not know this and could gain or lose a customer and or business partner. It's about the conversation, not the conversion.

And Now On To The Next Big Thing that will make you Rich?

Hey everyone,

I wanted to give a quick shout to make for SURE that you all listen to a call tonight from Brig Hart. I need to give some background for some of you that did not come in at the very first of this deal last March. yes, it has been a year in the making, but very worth the wait. I know for some of you it has been a wait and see and wait more and more, to the point of "so what's this time about". I can assure you that this is IT!

NETWORK MARKETING

As some background, Brig Hart is a man that is
the most successful network marketer in
History. He was in Amway for 10 years where
his team had 1 billion in sales, with him making
100 million. He then went to Monavie and his
team did a billion in sales in 3.5 years and he
once again made 100 million dollars, as well as
making lots of millionaires under him. He
retired from that, but felt like he wanted to
make 1 more run at 1 more venture. His vision
of a good run would be at a water product.

We originally were working with Earthwater. It
was a mineral loaded water with 70 trace
minerals and fulvic and humic properties. The
water is Black, but tastes like water. The
Benefits of the water were great with many
many testimonies of improved health issues.
Brig and Earthwater parted ways when there
were some contractual problems with them and
Earthwater was not doing things they had
agreed to do.

So that's when we went to Pure, which was going to help us get the water product (not Earthwater) going. After promising that they could do that, it did not materialize.

So, at this same time there was an international company 30 times the size of Pure that contacted Brig and pursued him wanting to be a part of this venture. The new water product is complete, and is a mineral water like Earthwater, only better.

We are moving forward at a very fast pace to come to market with this.

I will let you listen to the call from Brig tonight for specifics. But I will tell you that you will not want to miss out on this. Definitely worth the wait. There is a structure in place for making a great income on this water that will have wonderful health benefits to the consumer.

So, do you want to say: I have been waiting and waiting and this is just another plan that will not go anywhere, OR do you want to listen to the Plan of a man that has not only made himself and other multiple millions selling some great products, not once, but twice. Up to you and hope to see you there on the call.

Thanks

I have 2 short videos I want to show you guys about our new business venture. The first is a simple explanation of how you can make money in a very big hurry with this opportunity. The video that I will show you is a compensation plan from Jeunesse. The thing to remember is: the first scenario is starting with you and adding 2 the first month then in the next month those 2 add 2. then in the third month those 4 add 2 and so on until after 12 months you have 8188 people and 14, 315 dollars a month. Now this sounds great, but in our plan, it won't be just adding 2 people per level each month. We will be adding 2 people per level in 48 hours. So, in, if no glitches, then you should be at 15 levels which is approx. 163K a month. I know these numbers sound crazy, even the basic monthly build that is 14, 315 a month after 12 months is crazy, but this IS what we are talking about here folks. Brig and team have developed a new system that will allow you to build this team fast. The product is wonderful and sells itself. The new business plan will do the same. The plan will be on an app that you can show to someone in about 2 minutes flat. If they are interested, then you simply would connect 3-way calls with you, them, and CK. It really is this simple.

The second short video is an explanation about the Fulvic compounds that are in a water product. I don't think most of you have an inkling of a clue of the magnitude of this product and what it can do for you and others that you can help. Listen to this short video From Dr. Nuzum. He is a physician, and toxicologist and a professor, as well as a scientist and researcher. He has 7 doctorates. You will be amazed at the benefits of the fulvic acid that is in the new water product we have.

https://youtu.be/S2Bj5LgEbSl

https://youtu.be/vEqEEXB10lQ

Thanks

Afterword:

So, now where does this leave me with PURE?

I was skeptical in the beginning of this company, PURE, but, the quality and effectiveness of the product convinced me that PURE (www.livepure.com) has a solid product to back up the company's offering.

I have an Amazon membership which now costs me over $100 per year to belong to.

I use Amazon more than I would ever have believed a few years ago. I like it because they have what I want, when I want it and for a price, I'm happy to pay. I don't have to go to a store to be treated like I'm an inconvenience or disappointed when I can't find what it is, I came there to purchase.

PURE, is a $25 annual membership where I can source all my health and wellness needs which for now work for me!

At this time, I can tell you the business aspect of PURE does not work for me, but I will tell you this, it is working for many who have taken a chance on themselves to work for themselves and they are achieving some great results.

Now, there's this new venture with Brigg. If you get in early you may be one of the lucky ones who cashes in.

Will it work for you? Both company's products probably will. The business part, well that's up for you to decide. Only you know if your cut out for this business model. Most people aren't!

You are probably wondering why I wrote this? I did it so you can make an informed decision and counter the high-pressure tactics used by the majority of folks who believe in Network Marketing.

However, my intention was also to give you a comprehensive understanding of what is necessary to get into a business of your own.

The mainstream approach may be unrealistic for most regular folks who desire to own their own business.

Network Marketing is within the majorities reach if you are so inclined to take the plunge and take a chance on yourself.

It's up to you to make it work.

Good Luck,

Gary

9 781730 748769